Rosy Oliveira

Breastfeeding and neonatology

Rosy Oliveira

Breastfeeding and neonatology

Human milk extraction in neonatal units

ScienciaScripts

Imprint

Cover image: www.ingimage.com

This book is a translation from the original published under ISBN 978-620-6-75812-9.

Publisher:
Sciencia Scripts
is a trademark of
Dodo Books Indian Ocean Ltd. and OmniScriptum S.R.L publishing group

120 High Road, East Finchley, London, N2 9ED, United Kingdom
Str. Armeneasca 28/1, office 1, Chisinau MD-2012, Republic of Moldova, Europe
Printed at: see last page
ISBN: 978-620-7-62043-2

Contents

SUMMARY

INTRODUCTION: In addition to being the best food for babies, breast milk contributes to reducing infant mortality in children under five by up to 13%. Among the strategies to intensify breastfeeding and maintain lactation is the extraction of human milk in a neonatal environment. With the pandemic, new obstacles have arisen, such as the distancing of mothers in neonatal units, with repercussions for strategies to improve breastfeeding and maintain lactation in mothers of pre-term newborns, such as the reduction in milk extraction rates at the bedside in a neonatal environment. METHOD: This was an experience report study, using the Maguerez Arc methodology, at the Dr Cesar Cals General Hospital (HGCC), in Fortaleza/Ceara, from February to August 2022. RESULTS: In preterm newborns (PTNB), the mother's own milk should always be the first choice. With this in mind, the focus of the study was on strategies for maintaining lactation in mothers of preterm newborns, with an emphasis on bedside milk extraction. The associated factors were: Interruption of bedside milking, absence of a defined protocol, lack of staff awareness, overcrowding, difficulty in free access for mothers due to the worsening of the pandemic, absence of a place to support mothers, low professional adherence to training, low stock of pasteurised human milk for demand. Based on the aspects identified, a Standard Operating Procedure (SOP) was developed, as well as a milk extraction flow in a neonatal environment, meetings were held with the sectors involved, and training and awareness-raising were carried out with the teams, also involving the multi-professional residency. FINAL CONSIDERATIONS: With the control of the pandemic, it was possible to return to good practices that were not being carried out or that were reduced, such as milk extraction at the bedside in neonatal environments and skin-to-skin contact, but some support was needed to contribute to this return, such as training and sensitisation of professionals.

DESCRIPTORS

Breastfeeding; neonatology; COVID-19; premature newborn; lactation.

INTRODUCTION

Prematurity continues to cause public health concerns and accounts for the majority of perinatal morbidity and mortality, which can have repercussions in terms of immediate damage and late sequelae[1] . Among the most important strategies that significantly contribute to reducing the risks for this population is breastfeeding.

As well as being the best food for babies, breast milk contributes to reducing infant mortality in children under five by up to 13 per cent[2] , but it is still a challenge, especially in neonatal units.

With the aim of reducing neonatal mortality rates and improving care for newborns in maternity hospitals, the Ministry of Health (MoH) has set up the QualiNEO Strategy.

In neonatal units, one of the strategies to intensify breastfeeding and maintain lactation is breast stimulation and the extraction of human milk through bedside milking. This is a practice in which the mother expresses her milk next to her child's incubator or crib, and offers it to the newborn (NB) immediately after collection, under the supervision of a professional[3] .

During the pandemic, despite national recommendations to maintain breastfeeding and free access and stay in the neonatal unit for asymptomatic and non-contacting mothers[4] , the distancing had repercussions on the reduction of milk extraction at the bedside. Teams also need to reinvent themselves and develop strategies during challenging scenarios[5] .

Together with the high turnover of professionals and overcrowding in the units, there are potential factors that have had an impact on the practices of skin-to-skin contact, bedside milking and human milk donation.

Knowing the reality of the consequences of the pandemic and the indicators of the unit and developing targeted activities, such as sensitisation and training of professionals to encourage the maintenance of lactation of mothers of premature newborns through strategies such as bedside milking, encouraging skin-to-skin contact, stimulating the donation of human milk and promoting breastfeeding, it is possible to contribute to more babies receiving human milk, with the potential to reduce neonatal infections and mortality.

The aim of this study was to report on the experience of strategies and supports that favour the maintenance of lactation in mothers of premature newborns, with an emphasis on milk extraction at the bedside in neonatal units, using the Maguerez Arc method.

CHAPTER 1

PROFILE OF THE INSTITUTION AND THE MAGUEREZ ARC

The study was an experience report, using the Maguerez's Arc methodology, in a tertiary referral hospital for women's and children's health, located in Fortaleza/Ceara, from February to August 2022.

The hospital is a member of the QualiNEO Strategy and is a benchmark for the Human Milk Bank (HMB) and the Kangaroo Method (KM) in the state.

The institution has five neonatology units, two of which are NICUs (intensive care units), two NICU-CoUs (intermediate care units) and one NICU-CaU (kangaroo intermediate care units), with a total of 66 registered beds.

The units are staffed by neonatologists, nurses, nursing technicians, speech therapists, physiotherapists, among others, with employment contracts varying between civil servants (a minority) and cooperatives (the majority).

With regard to the Maguerez Arc, this can be defined as a problematisation methodology, collaborating in an educational-reflective process that contributes to the humanisation of care based on the experiences of the participants in their institution[6] .

The Maguerez Arc is made up of five stages: Observation of Reality; Key Points; Theorisation; Solution Hypothesis; Application to Reality[7] .

In the first stage, the researcher is encouraged to observe the context in which he or she is inserted and record the details, making it possible to identify the needs and define the problematisation.

The second stage is the search for possible causes and solutions. This stage is also known as defining the "key points".

In order to understand the origin of the difficulties and how to solve them, the third stage, theorising, is the search for knowledge, followed by the fourth stage, which is the formulation of hypotheses, in which the researchers begin to think more critically about possible solutions.

The fifth stage, applying reality, presents what has been developed and the decisions and answers found[7] .

"A CLOSER LOOK AT OUR REALITY"

The number of premature newborns in Brazil is significant. The country is among the ten in the world with the highest prematurity rates[8] .

As well as being the best food for babies, breast milk contributes to reducing infant mortality by up to 13% in children under five years of age[9] .

With the pandemic, new obstacles have become a concern in the current scenario, such as maintaining lactation in mothers of pre-term newborns.

The site of the current study was the neonatal units of a tertiary hospital in Fortaleza, Ceara, Brazil.

The hospital is a reference in Human Milk Banking and the Kangaroo Method in the state and has 02 neonatal intensive care units (NICU) with 20 beds, 02 conventional intermediate care units (CICU) with 36 beds and 01 conventional intermediate care unit (CICU) with 10 beds and 02 delivery rooms. These have a multi-professional team.

The hospital receives mothers from the municipality of Fortaleza and those referred from the state's high-risk prenatal centre.

The observation was carried out using the Neonatal Care Monitoring System (SMCON), the QualiNEO Strategy and medical records.

Through the Good Practices Portal, on the QualiNEO Platform, indicators for the year 2021 were evaluated. According to SMCON, skin-to-skin contact showed the following indicators: NBs < 1,500g: 1.82%; between 1,500 and 2,499g: 1.26%; > 2,500g: 1.87%.

With regard to the type of first enteral diet: < 1,500g: 14.02% colostrum, 12.80% pasteurised human milk (PHM), 0% formula and 1.83% no information (SI). Between 1,500g and 2,499g: 11.31% breast milk or colostrum, 3.52% LHP, 2.51% formula and 0.50% SI. > 2,500g: 13.92% breast milk or colostrum, 2.55% LHP, 5.26% formula and 0.85% SI.

With regard to the "diet prescribed at hospital discharge": 2,500g: breast milk 16.09%, breast milk and formula 31.23%, formula 19.24% and IS

17.35%. Skin-to-skin contact in the NICU or NICU was below the average of the other units participating in the QualiNEO strategy during the period evaluated.

Skin-to-skin contact is known to be one of the best ways of encouraging breastfeeding[10] . It is recommended to start feeding all newborn babies, preferably with raw or pasteurised breast milk, with the exception of those who are very unstable or have intestinal pathologies.

In PTNBs, the mother's own milk should always be the first choice[11] .

The focus of the study was therefore on strategies for maintaining lactation in mothers of premature newborns.

The pandemic has brought an even greater challenge in maintaining lactation for mothers of pre-term newborns. Together with the high turnover of professionals, overcrowding and lack of adherence to training, these are potential factors that interfere with the practices of skin-to-skin contact, bedside milking and human milk donation.

These supports need to be corrected and intensified, as well as standardising free access for parents to neonatal units, training and sensitising staff, discussing indicators and strategies involving infants.

Breastfeeding is undoubtedly the ideal nutrition for newborn babies, but it is still a challenge, especially in neonatal units. If there is no constant stimulation through breastfeeding to maintain milk production, breastfeeding can be compromised. One of the strategies in this case is breast stimulation. Awareness-raising among professionals, health education and support in the human milk extraction room can all help to maintain lactation in these mothers.

The distancing of mothers in neonatal units during the pandemic has had repercussions for many parents.

Despite national recommendations to maintain breastfeeding and free access and stay in the neonatal unit for asymptomatic and non-contacting mothers, institutional routines during the advance of the pandemic altered this routine[4] .

It is necessary for health professionals to advise mothers to perform constant milking as early as possible, even if their children are not yet feeding. They need to reinvent themselves and develop strategies in the current scenario.

Associated factors include: Interruption of bedside milking, lack of defined protocol, lack of staff awareness, overcrowding, difficulty in free access for mothers due to the worsening of the pandemic, lack of support facilities for mothers, low adherence of professionals to training, low stock of pasteurised human milk for demand.

Other major determinants are also present, such as socio-economic aspects related to the mothers' stay in the institution, the population's low adherence to human milk donation, and prematurity.

The prematurity and hospitalisation of PTNBs is already a challenge for maintaining breastfeeding. The pandemic has brought other difficulties.

Support to maintain lactation is necessary in the face of this current scenario.

In the next stage, it was decided to study some topics such as breastfeeding in neonatal units and the maintenance of lactation of these mothers will be studied in the course of this study, using the following descriptors: breastfeeding, breast feeding, lactancia materna; neonatologia, neonatology, neonatolog^a; COVID-19; recem- nascido prematuro, infant premature, recien nacido prematuro; lactapao, lactation, lactancia; metodo kangaroo, Kangaroo-Mother Care Method, Metodo Madre-Canguro.

"Reading and proposals to change our reality"

A search was carried out using established descriptors in databases such as Lilacs, as well as Google Scholar and Ministry of Health manuals.

Among the studies found, some were selected for use in theorising and contributing to the development of the instrument to be applied to professionals in neonatal units.

According to the selected literature. It is known that prematurity accounts for around 75% of neonatal mortality, with preterm babies being more susceptible to complications such as enterocolitis, sepsis, alterations in the neurological system, among others.

In order to reduce deaths in this population, the Ministry of Health has developed strategies such as the Baby-Friendly Hospital Initiative, the Kangaroo Method[12] and the Technical Standard Technical Procedures for Milking, Handling and Administering Raw Human Milk Exclusively from the Mother to the Child in the Neonatal Environment[3] .

Although breastfeeding is considered the best diet for newborn babies, especially preterm babies, there are factors that make breastfeeding difficult and contribute to early weaning for this population, such as stress, anxiety and worry among mothers of babies born prematurely[13] .

Despite the challenge, establishing breastfeeding is possible for a large proportion of premature newborns admitted to neonatal units.

This also requires trained professionals and the maintenance of good practices for children and families.

The institutions that are part of the Baby-Friendly Hospital Initiative have shown advantages in achieving these results[14] .

Other strategies to improve breastfeeding for preterm newborns are the Kangaroo Care Method (KMC), a nationally and internationally recognised public policy that contributes to good practice in neonatal health care and family care.

The breastfeeding process for mothers of newborns admitted to neonatal units begins with welcoming the family and helping them to stay with their children for as long as possible, making skin-to-skin contact as early as possible and manually expressing breast milk in order to maintain lactation.

The team that assists these women must be trained to welcome, guide and help them through this process[15] .

Studies show that there is a need for training for professionals in breastfeeding premature babies, including helping to guide the mothers of these babies.

In view of this and in continuity with the work being carried out, some hypotheses were raised that contributed to the development of a questionnaire using the google forms tool, to be applied to neonatal nursing professionals, also serving as a subsidy for on-site training and capacity building aimed at good neonatal care practices, with an emphasis on support that contributes to the promotion of breastfeeding in preterm infants.

Some of the questions served as a basis for the rest of the questionnaires, such as:

Have nursing professionals who work in neonatology already taken the Baby-Friendly Hospital Initiative Course (20-hour course)?

Have nursing professionals working in neonatology taken the Kangaroo Care Awareness Course?

✓ Are neonatal health professionals aware of the Technical Standard Technical Procedures for Milking, Handling and Administering Raw Human Milk Exclusively from Mother to Child in the Neonatal Environment?

Based on this, the following hypotheses were raised:

-1- There is a high turnover of professionals in neonatology and a significant number have not yet taken the recommended courses in good neonatal care practice;

-2- Due to overcrowding, neonatology professionals cannot be released to take the recommended courses;

-3- The pandemic has affected the practice of bedside milking due to the distance between mothers and neonatal units and it has not yet been normalised;

-4- Professionals lack knowledge of practices recommended and current;

-5- Strategies are needed to raise awareness of the development of good neonatal care practices.

Among the possible strategies already raised are:

✓ The IHAC and Kangaroo Method courses were held at different times in order to offer professionals more opportunities to take them;

✓ On-the-spot training is carried out ahead of bedside milking;

✓ Construction of Standard Operating Procedures for the Milking, Handling and Administration of Raw Human Milk Exclusively from Mother to Child in the Neonatal Environment, Colostrum Therapy and Translactation;

✓ Intensifying and supporting activities with more premature newborns, among others.

CHAPTER 2

Stages of the Maguerez Arc

Preparation of Stage I - Observation of reality.

The observation was carried out by consulting the database of the Neonatal Care Monitoring System (SMCON), through the Good Practices Portal, on the QualiNEO Platform, using data related to breastfeeding and observing the period from January to December 2021.

SMCON is a platform for monitoring the indicators monitored by the QualiNEO Strategy, which is regularly fed by the participating institutions and the Fernandes Figueira Institute (IFF).

According to SMCON, in 2021, the hospital studied registered 204 NBs, admitted to neonatology, weighing <1,500g; 480 NBs weighing between 1,500 and 2,499g; 691 NBs weighing >2,500g.

With regard to those who made skin-to-skin contact in neonatal inpatient units, the unit studied had significantly lower than average adherence than the other units that are part of the monitoring system.

According to the register of newborns registered in SMCON at the institution, only 4 (1.96%) weighing < 1,500g, 7 (1.46%) weighing between 1,500g and 2,499g and 11 (1.59%) > 2, 500g had a record of

skin-to-skin contact in the first stage of the kangaroo method.

Studies have shown that skin-to-skin contact is one of the best ways of encouraging breastfeeding and facilitating a good start[8] .

With regard to the type of first enteral diet administered, distributed by weight, it was also observed that the institution was below the average referenced by the other QualiNEO Strategy units (Graph 1), in the supply of human milk, which motivated this work and support for the return and improvement of related good neonatal practices.

It should be noted that the hospital has experienced a period of challenges in terms of collecting and entering data into the platform, which has had repercussions in terms of faulty records in the system.

Graph 1. Human milk offered as the first enteral diet, distributed by weight of NBs registered at the unit, Fortaleza, Ceara, Brazil, 2021.

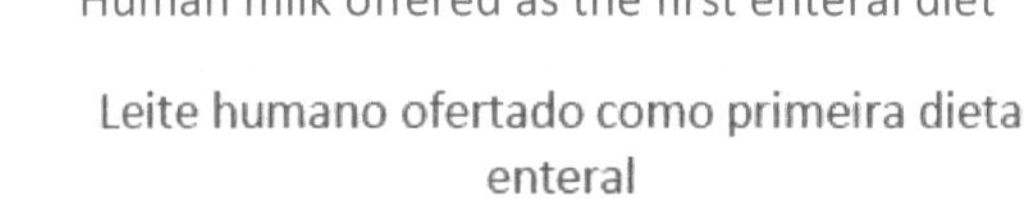

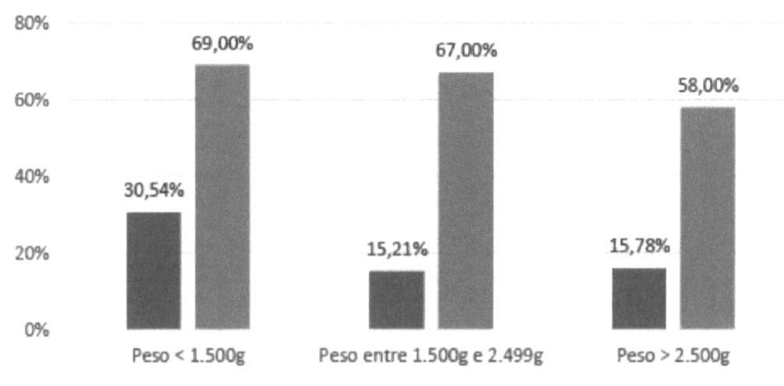

■ Oferta de Leite humano na instituição

■ Oferta de leite humano nas unidades QualiNEO

■ Human milk supply in the institution

■ Supply of human milk in QualiNEO units

Among the registered newborns weighing <1,500g, only 62 (30.54%) had a record of an enteral diet using human milk, either raw or pasteurised. In those between 1,500g and 2,499g there were 73 (15.21%) and in those > 2,500g there were 109 (15.78%).

It is known that breast milk is the most important food for newborns due to its nutritional value and biological complexity, especially for PTNBs[9] .

With regard to "Diet prescribed at hospital discharge" (Graph 2), among the 93 NBs discharged from the institution weighing <1,500g, 42

(45.16%) were prescribed human milk at discharge from the unit neonatal. Of the 311 weighing between 1,500g and 2,499g, 164 (52.73 per cent)

found prescribed human milk. In those > 2,500g there were 166 (46.24%).

Graph 2. Diet prescribed at discharge from the neonatal unit with human milk, distributed by weight of NBs registered at the unit, Fortaleza, Ceara, Brazil, 2021.

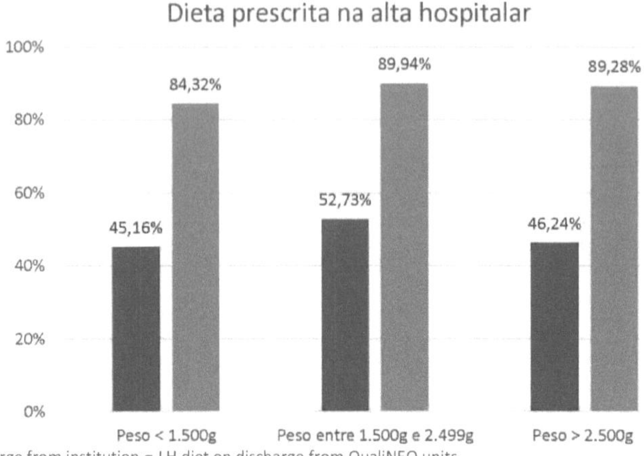

In addition to the pandemic, other factors may have contributed to these results, such as the fragile relationship, since most of the professionals are from cooperatives, which has repercussions on high turnover.

Stage 2: Preparation of Stage II - Key Points

At the start of Stage II, the following questions were answered:

"What in the reality of your experience is lacking, inconsistent or worrying?"

The answer was: Consequences of the pandemic on the maintenance of lactation in mothers of preterm newborns.

Another question was: "What needs to be corrected, resolved, improved or modified in the scenario?", and the following answers were given:

-1- Return to bedside milking; Intensify skin-to-skin contact;

-2- Encourage the donation of human milk; Standardise free access for parents to neonatal units;

-3- Train and sensitise staff (Baby-Friendly Hospital Initiative (BFHI), MC, Good Neonatal Care Practices);

-4- Discuss indicators; encourage the maintenance of lactation in the Human Milk Extraction Room.

With the responses, some points were defined to be addressed:

✓ COVID-19 pandemic;

✓ Overcrowding;

✓ High turnover of professionals;

✓ Lack of incentives/conditions for professionals to attend training sessions;

✓ Lack of Standard Operating Procedure and Flow;

permanent *on-site* education.

Preparation of Stage III - Theorisation

It is known that prematurity accounts for around 75 per cent of neonatal mortality and that this population is more susceptible to complications.

In order to reduce mortality, the Ministry of Health has developed strategies such as the Baby-Friendly Hospital Initiative, the Kangaroo Method[10] and the Technical Standard Technical Procedures for Milking, Handling and Administering Raw Human Milk Exclusively from Mother to Child in the Neonatal Environment.

Other strategies to improve breastfeeding for preterm newborns are the Kangaroo Method, which has national coverage and international recognition, and is a public policy that contributes to good practice in neonatal health care and family care.

It is known that skin-to-skin contact is an important strategy that contributes to breastfeeding[8] .

The breastfeeding process for mothers of newborns admitted to neonatal units begins with welcoming the family. The team that cares for these women must be trained to welcome, guide and assist them in this process[11] .

It is recommended to start feeding within the first 24 hours of life, preferably with raw or pasteurised breast milk, for all newborn babies, with the exception of those who are very unstable or have intestinal pathologies that contraindicate it.

In PTNBs, the mother's own milk should always be the first choice[9] . With this in mind, the focus of the study was on strategies for maintaining lactation in mothers of premature newborns, with an emphasis on bedside milk extraction.

Preparation of Stage IV - Solution Hypotheses

Based on what has been presented, the following solution hypotheses have been raised:

✓ Construction of a Standard Operating Procedure (SOP) for Technical Procedures for the Milking, Handling and Administration of Exclusive Raw Human Milk from Mother to Child in the Neonatal Environment, Colostrum Therapy and Translactation, and a Flow Chart for the Extraction of Milk at the Bedside;

✓ *On-site* training on bedside milking;

✓ The BFHI and Kangaroo Method courses were held at different times in order to offer professionals more opportunities to take them;

✓ Intensify and support activities with mothers of premature newborns.

Preparation and Application of Stage V - Application to reality

The study showed that awareness-raising strategies are needed to develop good neonatal care practices aimed at breastfeeding. Milking at the bedside in neonatal units was already a practice, but with the pandemic and the distancing of mothers, it was discontinued.

One of the initial supports was to develop a Standard Operating Procedure (SOP) and a Flow for organising the ward, which had not existed until then. These were discussed at a meeting between representatives of neonatology, the human milk bank, the delivery room and the rooming-in unit.

Training and sensitisation sessions were then held with professionals. Some had not yet experienced the practice, as it had been suspended during the pandemic.

Due to the significant turnover in the sector, there were employees who were unfamiliar with the technique. Health education sessions were held with professionals and with the residency, a great support in the institution.

Among the 10 steps for neonatal care, in addition to Step 4, which is "Feed the NB as early as possible and preferably with breast/human milk", Step 7 includes "Practise the Kangaroo Method and integrate the entire multi-professional team in individualised care".

After developing the action plan and building strategies, training and awareness-raising activities were started for milk extraction in the neonatal environment and also to intensify skin-to-skin contact in these units, which was again interrupted by the increase in covid-19 cases at the beginning of this year.

Sessions were held with neonatology and residency professionals to discuss skin-to-skin contact and bedside milking in order to intensify good practice through guidance, awareness-raising, clarification of doubts, discussion of standard operating procedures, flow, statistics spreadsheets, etc.

In addition to expressing human milk in a neonatal environment, some topics that contribute to or bring results related to maintaining lactation in premature newborns were emphasised during the training sessions. These include

-1- QualiNEO Strategy;

-2- Obstetric and Neonatal Care Monitoring System and its related indicators;

-3- Kangaroo method;

-4- Free access for parents;

-5- Reception, support and breastfeeding support;

-6- Technical note on bedside milking, SOP and flow developed;

-7- Spreadsheet for monitoring the extraction of human milk in the neonatal unit;

-8- Importance of the HICC and MC courses.

The BFHI and MC courses also emphasised the importance of lactation maintenance for the mothers of PTNBs and bedside milk extraction in neonatal units.

In the *on-site* training sessions, it was noted that some professionals had only recently joined the service and had not learnt the bedside milking practice that used to take place before the pandemic.

There was also a lack of knowledge among professionals about the app and its benefits, making it necessary to carry out a situational diagnosis in order to continue the support that will help to intensify good practice.

With this in mind, a checklist was developed to be applied in the courses offered by the neonatology department and in training programmes to guide support.

In order to monitor this, and with the support of the neonatology nursing coordinators, the neonatal units were instructed to fill in the Manual Bedside Milking Extraction form again.

As it was identified during the QualiNEO Strategy monitoring meetings that the completeness of the institution's data was also below the average for the state, from August onwards neonatology appointed a nurse to help with the Neonatal and Obstetric Care Monitoring System forms.

CONCLUSION

Despite the importance of strategies to promote breastfeeding and maintain lactation for mothers of premature newborns admitted to the neonatal ward, there are challenges in consolidating these practices, which has been intensified during the Covid-19 pandemic.

Prematurity and the hospitalisation of PTNBs is already a challenge for maintaining breastfeeding. The pandemic has had repercussions that have led to mothers distancing themselves from neonatal units and thus reducing skin-to-skin contact, milk collection at the bedside, and the frequency of visits to the collection room of human milk banks, reflecting on the indicators presented.

With the control of the pandemic, it was possible to return to good practices that were not being carried out or that had been reduced, such as the extraction of milk at the bedside in neonatal environments, but some support was needed to contribute to this return, such as training and sensitisation of professionals.

By using the Maguerez's Arc, we had the opportunity to develop reflective-scientific thinking and maintain an organised approach to defining the difficulties encountered and contributing to strategies to improve the maintenance of lactation in mothers of newborns admitted to neonatal units, such as milk extraction at the bedside.

As it is still a challenge, strategies remain in place and others still need to be developed to direct support towards good practices that contribute to maintaining breastfeeding.

REFERENCES

1 . Adriano, AP, Souta, ES, Lopes, LS, Santos, ML, Lobato, MV, Sanches, RP. Neonatal mortality related to prematurity. [Internet]. Res., Soc. Dev. 2021. V 11 (4). [cited 2022set16]. Available at: https://rsdjournal.org/index.php/rsd/article/view/21565.

2 Ministry of Health (BR). Campaign encourages breastfeeding in Brazil. [Internet]. Rio de Janeiro: Fiocruz. [cited 2022 Sep 05]. Available at:<https://www.bio.fiocruz.br/index.php/br/noticias/2542-campanha-encourages breastfeeding in brazil.

3 Ministry of Health (BR). Technical procedures for milking, handling and administering raw human milk exclusively from mothers to their own children in a neonatal environment. Technical Note. Brasilia: HMB Network, 2017.

4 Ministry of Health (BR). Newborn Care in times of the COVID-19 pandemic: Recommendations for the Kangaroo Method: Recommendations for the kangaroo method during the COVID-19 pandemic. Rio de Janeiro: Fiocruz. 2020.

5 Dantas, AC, Santos, W, Nascimento, AA, Lorraynne AM. Reflecting on the context of breastfeeding during the COVID-19 pandemic. Enferm. Foco. 2020; 11 (Esp. 2): 236-239.

6 Borille, DC, Brusamarello, T, Paes, RP, Mazza, VA, Lacerda, MR et al. The application of the Maguerez arc method of problematisation in data collection in nursing research: an experience report. Texto Contexto Enferm.2012; 21 (1): 209-216.

7. Colombo AA, Berbel, NA. The methodology of problematisation with the Maguire Arch and its relationship with teachers' knowledge. Semina: Social and Human Sciences. 2007; 28 (2): 121-146.

8. Chawanpaiboon S, Vogel JP, Moller AB, Lumbiganon P, Petzold M, Hogan D, et al. Global, regional, and national estimates of levels of preterm birth in 2014: a systematic review and modelling analysis.

Lancet Glob Health. 2019; 7(1):e37-46. https://doi.org/10.1016/S2214-109X(18)30451-0.

9. Brazil, Ministry of Health. All for breastfeeding: Campaign encourages breastfeeding in Brazil. The Ministry of Health recommends breastfeeding until the age of 2 or more and exclusively for the first six months of life. 2021. Available at: < https://www.gov.br/pt-br/noticias/saude-e-vigilancia-sanitaria/2021/07/campanha-incentiva-o aleitamento-materno-no-brasil>.

10. Widstrom, AM, Brimdyr, K., Svensson, K., Cadwell, K, Nissen, E. Skin-to-skin contact the first hour after birth, underlying implications and clinical practice. Acta Pediatr. 2019; Available from: <108:1192-204. DOI: 10.1111/apa.14754>. Accessed on: 15 May 2022.

11. Villela, LD, Moreira, ME. Nutritional Protocol for the Neonatal Unit. Rio de Janeiro: Fiocruz, Fernandes Figueira National Institute for Women's, Children's and Adolescents' Health, 2020. 39p .: il. Available at: < https://doi.org/10.1590/1983-1447.2019.20180406>. Accessed May 2022.

12. Cunha, G, Rodrigues, FA, Herber, S. Breastfeeding of premature infants in a child-friendly hospital. Sao Paulo: Revista Recien. 2020; 10(30):168-Breastfeeding of premature infants in a child-friendly hospital.

13. Euzebio, BL, Lanzarini, TB, Americo GD, Pessota, CU, Cicollela, DA, - Fioravante Junior, GA, Kasmirscki, C. Breastfeeding: difficulties encountered by mothers that contribute to early weaning. Boletim da Saude, Porto Alegre, v. 26, n. 2, p. 83-90 jul./dez. 2017. Available at https://docs.bvsalud.org/biblioref/2020/10/1121329/8390.pdf. Accessed on 20 May 2023.

14. LIMA, A. P. et al. Exclusive breastfeeding of premature infants and reasons for its interruption in the first month after hospital discharge. Revista Gaucha de Enfermagem, Porto Alegre, v. 40, e20180406, 2019.

Available at: https://seer.ufrgs.br/ index.php/rgenf/article/view/96147. Accessed on: 10 June 2022.

15. Ministry of Health (BR). Secretariat for Health Care. Department of Strategic Programme Support. Humanised newborn care: Kangaroo method: technical manual. 3. ed. - BrasHia: Ministerio da Saude, 2017. 340 p.: ill.

Annexes

Annex 1: Standard Operating Procedure

QUALITY MANAGEMENT	
Document Type:	COD: POP.00
STANDARD OPERATING PROCEDURE	DATE: 00/00/0000 VERSE:
Document title:	
Milking, Handling and Administering Raw Human Milk Exclusively from Mother to Child in a Neonatal Setting	

WHO:	Nursing team
WHEN:	Daily
WHERE:	Neonatal Units

NECESSARY CONDITIONS	
Materials	**Documents and Systems**
· Beanie · Masks · Safety goggles · Procedure gloves · Soap and water or hand sanitiser · 70% alcohol · Gazes · Standardised graduated sterile cup	· Clinical Monitoring Sheet Neonatal · Milking Control Spreadsheet Bedside

DESCRIPTION OF THE PROCEDURE
• Welcome the mother and explain the procedure; • Hand hygiene. Professionals should follow the hand-washing recommendations for health services. Mothers should remove ornaments, fasten their

hair and put on a cap and mask, sanitising hands up to elbow height with soap and water;

• Make sure you stop. Professionals should use recommended PPE. Provide a suitable area and sanitise with 70% alcohol;

• Provide a standardised graduated sterile cup and gauze;

• Encourage the mother to massage the whole breast, in an areola-thorax direction, performing circular movements. If she can't, a professional can help her. Advise her to avoid talking, sneezing or coughing while milking.

- Guide/position the thumb on the upper edge of the areola and the other fingers on the lower edge (base of the breast), gently pressing and releasing several times. Dispose of the first drops of milk in sterile gauze to be discarded;
- Pour the milked milk into the cup provided and then into the syringe for gavage, under the supervision of the nursing staff;
- Give raw milked human milk (LHOC) to the recipient immediately after collection, respecting the medical prescription for volume and route of administration;
- In the event of surplus LHOC, sanitise the bottle with 70% alcohol, identify it with the mother's full name, date and time of collection and immediately send it in an isothermal box with recyclable ice to the Human Milk Bank for immediate freezing;
- Remove gloves and sanitise hands;
- After administration, the nursing professional who carried out the procedure should record the amount given, according to the medical prescription, on the Neonatal Clinical Monitoring Sheet and the Bedside Milking Control Sheet.
- Encourage mothers to return to milk at the bedside during diet times when they are in hospital and to attend the Human Milk Bank during breaks, stimulating the breasts and milking for the times when they are unable to be in the institution. Periodically expressing human milk and donating it should be encouraged whenever possible.

EXPECTED RESULTS:

- Offering raw milked human milk to neonates immediately after collection;
- Contribution to maintaining lactation.

IN THE EVENT OF NON-COMPLIANCE:

If any non-compliance is identified in the human milk to be offered, do not administer.

REFERENCES

1. BRAZIL. Ministry of Health. Secretariat for Health Care. Department of Strategic Programme Support. Humanised newborn care: Kangaroo method : technical manual / Ministry of Health, Secretariat of Health Care, Department of Strategic Programmatic Support. - 3. ed. - Brasilia: Ministry of Health, 2017.
2. BRAZIL, Ministry of Health. Technical procedures for milking, handling and administering raw human milk exclusively from mothers to their own children in a neonatal environment. Technical Note. Brasilia: HMB Network, 2017.
3. CARVALHO, M. R. Amamentapao: Bases CienHficas - 4 ed. Rio de Janeiro:

Guanabara Koogan, 2017.

Annex 2: Milking, Handling and Administration of Raw Human Milk from Mother to Child in a Neonatal Setting

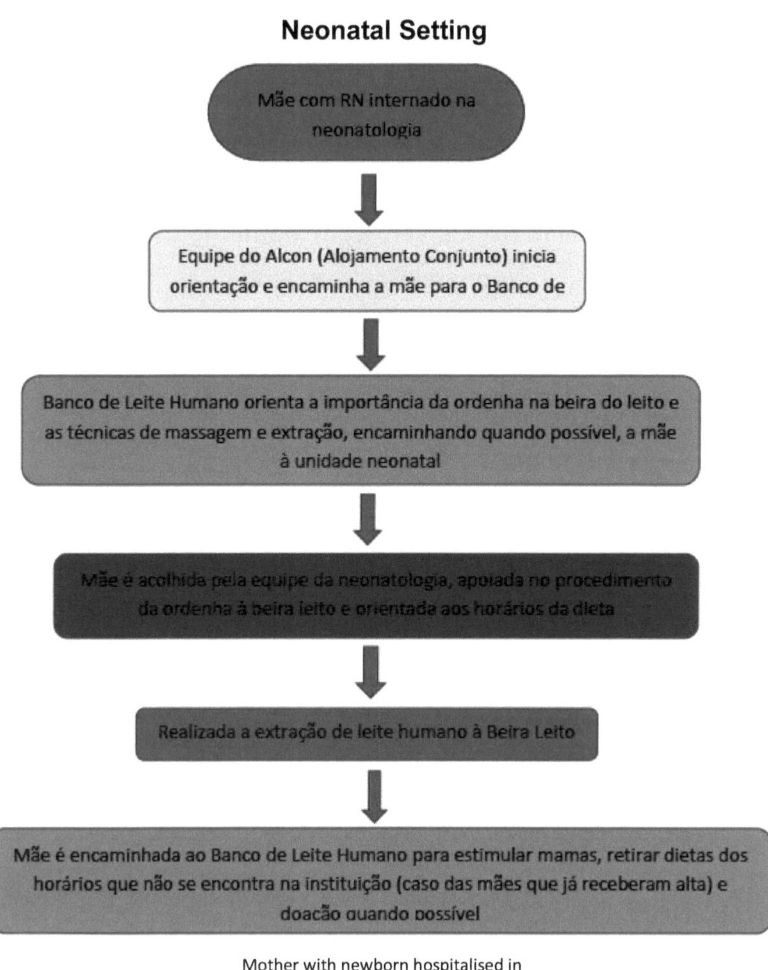

Mother with newborn hospitalised in neonatology

Alcon team (Joint Accommodation) begins counselling and refers the mother to the

The Human Milk Bank provides guidance on the importance of milking at the bedside and on massage and extraction techniques, referring the mother to the neonatal unit when possible.

Mother is welcomed by the neonatology team, supported in the procedure milking procedure at the bedside and instructed on diet times

Bedside human milk extraction carried out

The mother is sent to the Human Milk Bank to stimulate the breasts, remove the diets from the when she is not in the institution (in the case of mothers who have already been discharged) and donation when possible

Annex 3: Check List Milking, Handling and Administration of Raw Human Milk Exclusively from Mother to Child in the Neonatal Environment

On-site training

Name: Date:

Category/Function:Unit:

1. How long have you been with the organisation?

( ) More than 10 years ago

( ) Between 5 and 10 years

( ) Between 2 and 5 years

( ) Between 1 and 2 years

( ) Under 1 year old

2. Have you already taken the IHAC course?

Yes ( ) No ( )

3. Have you already taken the Kangaroo Method course?

Yes ( ) No ( )

4. Do you know what bedside milking is? Yes ( ) No ( )

5. Do you perform or identify bedside milking in your facility?

( ) yes, always ( ) I watched before the pandemic ( ) I watch less often than before the pandemic ( ) rarely ( ) sometimes ( ) no, never ( ) Other:

6. Do you know the standard operating procedure and flow of bedside extraction?

( ) yes, both ( ) only one ( ) none

7. Do you guide and encourage mothers in your unit to perform bedside extraction?

Yes ( ) No ( )

8. In your opinion, what are the benefits of bedside milking?
9. What do you see as the biggest challenges in performing bedside milking?
10. What do you suggest to intensify bedside milking in your unit?

Annex 4: Check List Skin-to-skin Training and Beira Milking Bed

-1- QualiNEO Strategy;

-2- Obstetric and neonatal care monitoring system;

-3- Related indicators;

-4- The Kangaroo Method as a Health Policy and Perinatal Care Model;

-5- Kangaroo position: advantages, public, roles of the health team: 1[a] stage: pregnancy, NICU, NICU.

-6- Free access for parents, reception, support and breastfeeding support;

-7- Breastfeeding: Bedside milking, Technical note, SOP and flow;

-8- Manual milk extraction technique;

-9- Spreadsheet for monitoring the extraction of human milk in the neonatal unit;

-10- Importance of taking the BFHI course (all professionals who work with mothers and babies should take it) and MC;

-11- Reinforcing the importance of recording the first skin-to-skin contact and filling in the volume of milk on the bedside milking indicator sheet.

Technical Procedures for Milking, Handling and Administering Raw Human Milk Exclusively from Mother to Child in the Neonatal Environment

Source: National Reference Centre for Human Milk Banks - Fernandes Figueira Institute / Oswaldo Cruz Foundation / Ministry of Health

Authors: Danielle Aparecida da Silva, Nicole Oliveira Mota Gianini, Mariana Simoes, Jonas Borges da Silva, Joao Aprigio Guerra de Almeida, Franz Reis Novak, Miriam Oliveira dos Santos, Virginia Beatrizde Resende Silva, Andrea Penha-Spinola Fernandes.

Key words: Raw Human Milk, Neonatology, Donor, Premature.

SUMMARY

1. Presentation

Technical Procedures for Milking, Handling and Administering Raw Human Milk Exclusively from Mother to Child in a Neonatal Setting

With the evolution of techniques, processes and equipment, neonatal units have been keeping smaller and smaller babies alive and the nutrition of these infants has become a challenge. The best food for the newborn is the mother's own milk, according to the consensus of the world's literatureL In view of this, the Global Network of Human Milk Banks (rBLH) has issued guidelines for the collection of milk from the mother in the neonatal environment, in order to offer the best food for the sick newborn, aid their recovery and favour the maintenance of breastfeeding. Studies show that when we milk at the bedside, with the mother seeing or in close contact with the newborn, there is an increase in the volume of human milk milked. This standard offers the possibility of creating a routine for the use of raw milked human milk (LHOC), offering intact protective factors such as immunoglobulins, lactoferrin, peroxidase and others, as well as the balanced formation of the microbiome, with less chance of bacterial translocation and sepsis. But we mustn't forget that this newborn is extremely vulnerable, so recommendations must be followed to minimise or extinguish any risk inherent in the process.

This publication is aimed at healthcare professionals to ensure the handling and use of LHOc in the neonatal hospital environment, with a view to patient safety. The document contains guidelines for obtaining hygienic and sanitary LHOC, with the main focus on the possible risks inherent in its milking, storage, preservation, transport, portioning and administration in the hospital environment (Neonatal Intensive Care Units - NICU,

Conventional Intermediate Neonatal Care Unit - UCINCO, Kangaroo Intermediate Neonatal Care Unit - UCINCA, Joint Accommodation -ALCON, Maternal ICU, milking parlours (SLO), human milk collection point (PCLH) and human milk bank (BLH).]

2. Objective

This standard establishes the processes for milking, storing, preserving, transporting, portioning and administering raw human milk, exclusively from the mother to her own child, in a neonatal environment, with a view to the quality of breast milk, food and nutritional safety and the maintenance of breastfeeding.

3. Complementary Documents

RDC 171 of 2006 - Standards for the Operation of Human Milk Banks

Ordinance MS 930/2012 - Guidelines and Objectives for the organisation of comprehensive and humanised care for the critically ill or potentially critically ill newborn and the criteria for classifying and qualifying Neonatal Unit beds within the scope of the Unified Health System (SUS).

BLH-IFF/NT09.04- Donors: Screening, Selection and Follow-up. 2004

BLH-IFF/NT 11.04- Hygiene and Conduct: Employees

BLH-IFF/NT 12.04- Hygiene and Conduct: Donors

BLH-IFF/NT 14.04- Hygiene and Conduct: Environment

BLH-IFF/NT 16.04- Milking: Hygienic and sanitary procedures. 2004

BLH-IFF/NT 17.04- Labelling of Raw Milked Human Milk

BLH-IFF/NT 18.04 - Pre-storage of Raw Milked Human Milk

<u>Technical Procedures for Milking, Handling and Administering Raw Human Milk Exclusively from Mother to Child in the</u> Neonatal <u>Environment</u>

BLH-IFF/NT 19.04-Transport of LHO. 2004

BLH-IFF/NT 20.04 - Temperature Control of Isothermal Boxes

BLH-IFF/NT 24.04 - Defrosting Raw Human Milk

BLH-IFF/NT 38.04 - Temperature Control of Freezers. 2004

BLH-IFF/NT 39.04 - Temperature Control of Refrigerators. 2004

BLH-IFF/NT 41.04 - Distribution of Milked Human Milk.2004

BLH-IFF/NT 43.04 - Care for the Handling of Milked Human Milk in a Hospital Environment. 2004

BLH-IFF/NT 44.04 - Control of Thermometers. 2004

4. Definitions

For the purposes of this Standard, the following definitions apply:

4.1. Biosafety: a set of measures aimed at preventing, minimising or eliminating risks inherent in research, production, teaching, technological development and service provision activities, with a view to the health of humans, animals, the preservation of the environment and the quality of the results.

4.2. Good Handling Practices for Milked Human Milk: a set of guidelines that must be observed when handling human milk in order to guarantee its quality.

4.3. Cold chain: the condition in which chilled or frozen products must be kept, under control and registration, from collection to consumption, with the aim of preventing the erosion of the myriobiota and promoting changes in their composition.

4.4. Hygienic and sanitary conditions: conditions established to guide and standardise procedures, with the aim of ensuring the quality of the process from the point of view of public health.

4.5. Packaging: the environment in which the product is stored, in such a way as to guarantee the maintenance of its biological value without harming the environment.

4.6. Standardised Packaging for Milked Human Milk: packaging tested and validated by a competent body, used for packaging milked human milk, observing all the requirements established for this purpose.

4.7. Storage: temperature and time conditions under which the pasteurised product is kept until it is consumed.

Technical Procedures for Milking, Handling and Administering Raw Human Milk Exclusively from Mother to Child in a Neonatal Setting

4.8. Diet Registration Form: a control sheet with information about the collection, the volume of human milk offered to the Newborn, the person responsible for the process, which must be filled in after the collection of human milk. See o Annex to this Standard.

4.9. Infant: child aged up to 24 months.

4.10. Milked Human Milk: the name given to human milk obtained through the milking procedure.

4.11. Raw Human Milk: the name given to milked human milk that has not yet undergone the pasteurisation process.

4.12. Non-conformity: failure to meet established quality requirements.

4.13. Nursing mother: a term used to refer to a woman who is breastfeeding.

4.14. Milking: refers to the extraction of the mother's **milk** secretion.

4.15. Pre-storage: storage, under suitable thermal conditions, of milked human milk before pasteurisation.

4.16. Recipients: customers who need the products supplied by the Milk Banks.

4.17. Labelling: the process of indicating the contents of a container or bottle by applying a label which, however, is not an integral part of it.

4.18. Maximum and minimum thermometers: instruments designed to measure internal or external temperatures, recording their maximum and minimum values over a given period of time.

5. General Considerations

5.1. O access to collection/manipulation areas should be restricted to the personnel directly involved.

5.2. All employees involved in the handling of human milk must be trained in personal hygiene practices, in accordance with ICHC standards, and be equipped with equipment (cap, mask, glove, glasses) to ensure the protection of human milk and meet biosafety requirements (see BLH- IFF/NT 15.04 - Biosafety).

Technical Procedures for Milking, Handling and Administering Raw Human Milk Exclusively from Mother to Child in a Neonatal Setting

5.3. All employees should be instructed and encouraged to report to their immediate superiors any conditions relating to the environment, equipment or personnel, especially skin, respiratory or gastrointestinal tract diseases, which they consider harmful to the quality of human milk.

5.4. The nursing mother should be instructed in personal hygiene practices, according to the ICHR, and given information on good milk handling practices.

human milk (see BLH-IFF/NT - 16.04 - Milking: Hygienic and sanitary procedures) to collect the milk.

5.5. The staff member in charge must be able to answer any questions the nursing mother may have during the newborn's hospitalisation at the time of milk collection.

5.6. Milking must take place in environments with satisfactory hygiene and sanitary conditions (see BLH-IFF/NT 14.04 - Hygiene and Conduct: Environment), free from risk factors that could lead to non-conformities in the milked human milk.

5.7. The use of accessories (watches, bracelets, rings, etc.) and products that may smell (perfumes, creams, etc.) should be discouraged for both donors and employees (see NR 32).

5.8. The administration of raw human milk from the mother to her child should preferably take place immediately after collection.

5.9. In order to preserve the quality of the product at the time of consumption, the handling of human milk in a hospital environment must

observe the recommendations for this purpose set out in BLH-IFF/NT Standard 43.04 - Care in the Handling of Milked Human Milk

Ambiente Hospitalar, 2004.

Technical Procedures for Milking, Handling and Administering Raw Human Milk Exclusively from Mother to Child in the Neonatal Environment

6. Routines

6.1. Breast massage

№	AGENT	AQAO	OBSERVATION	COMMENTS
01	Employee	Put on a cap and mask. Hand hygiene according to the protocol adopted by the institution's ICHR.	Minimises the risk of contamination of raw human milk	
02	Employee	Use personal protective equipment (goggles and procedure gloves) that allows for the safe handling of human milk, in accordance with the protocol adopted by the institution's HICC.		As well as protecting employees individually, it minimises the risk of contaminating human milk.
03	Mae	Remove ornaments, tie up your hair and cover it with a cap and		

		put on a mask.		
04	Mae	Carry out hand hygiene in accordance with the specific protocol for this purpose, adopted by the Institution's CCIH.		
05	Employee	Explain why massage is performed before milking	Massage helps the breast to empty evenly and improves the milk letdown reflex.	Never start milking without prior massage.
06	Employee	Welcome the mother, massage her back to stimulate the oxytocin reflex.	Improves milk ejection reflex	

Technical Procedures for Milking, Handling and Administering Exclusive Mother-to-Child Human Milk in the Neonatal Environment

07	Employee/Mother	Encourage the mother to massage the whole breast, in the direction of the areola to the thorax, making circular movements; if she can't, a professional can help her.	Improves milk mobilisation. Strong pressure can traumatise the breasts.	Use a flat hand. Do not press hard . I've always supported my mum.
08	Mae	Recline slightly forwards		
09	Employee/Mother	Hold the lower part of the breasts while rocking them slowly	Facilitates the ejection reflex.	

6.2. Milking

Both manual and mechanical milking, following the guidelines below, can be carried out in the NICU, NICU, NACU, ALCON, maternal hospitalisation unit.

Milking - Additional site considerations

Intensive Care - O staff member will assist the nursing mother, following the technical recommendations for milking. At the end of the milking process, the properly labelled milk will be used immediately or sent for storage under refrigeration or freezing.

Conventional Intermediate Unit-Milking will be carried out for those NBs who eventually suckle at the breast, but who need milk afterwards; premature babies who get tired before they are satisfied; and those who receive milk by cup. The milking technique must follow manual milking routines and be supervised by the Conventional Intermediate Unit team.

Intermediate Kangaroo Unit - The collection will be carried out so that the baby's milk is given raw, according to the doctor's prescription, immediately after milking. Guided and supervised by the NICU team, following the technical recommendations for manual milking.

Joint Accommodation - LHOC can help maintain breastfeeding in cases of cleft breast, where a break from breastfeeding can help recovery, difficulty latching on, breast engorgement and other situations.

Technical Procedures for Milking, Handling and Administering Raw Human Milk Exclusively from Mother to Child in a Neonatal Environment

Maternal hospitalisation unit - some situations prevent the mother from travelling to the neonatal unit, SCLH, PCLH, BLH. In order to maintain breastfeeding and offer the best food for the newborn, LHOC collection can be carried out in this environment following the guidelines below.

Introduce the mother to the different milking methods available in the parlour, allowing her to try them out, while observing the correct technique; the choice of milking method should be left up to the mother. For immediate consumption, it would be ideal to start milking 15 or 20 minutes before administration. Don't overvalue one method over another.

6.3. Manual milking

№	AGENT	THE CAO	NOTE	COMMENTS
01	Mae	Clean the breasts. a. Clean the breasts with gas and water potable or; b. Wash breasts and nipples with clean water current or; c. Use your own human milk after the elimination of the first jets.	It reduces the risk of contamination and also aims to minimise the occurrence of scaling.	Do not use soap or any other type of sanitising product. Do not use creams or ointments with moisturising properties.
02	Employee	Make it available: A. Inert and indecisively sterile container with a wide mouth and a plastic lid that allows for perfect closure, easy to clean and resistant to sterilisation, with a volume compatible with the mother's milk production, with a label to be filled in. B. Or sterile syringe with sealed tip with a sterile device.		The sterile containers should now be refrigerated in the cool box.

Technical Procedures for Milking, Handling and Administering Raw Human Milk Exclusively from Mother to Child in the Neonatal Environment

03	Employee	Provide a support table, previously sanitised in accordance with the protocol adopted by the Institution's		

		ICHR.		
04	Employee/Mother	Massage the breasts - according to item 6.1.1		Teaching massage techniques
05	Employee/Mother	Homeexpression softening the areola		
06	Employee	Label the sterile container with the name of the recipient's mother, date and time of collection.	The label must be resistant to humidity and cooling and will not fade when wet.	
07	Employee/Mother	Open the container and place the lid with the sterile side facing upwards on a table. In the case of direct syringe extraction, keep the embolus protected inside the packaging.		
08	Employee/Mother	Place the thumb on the upper edge of the areola and the other fingers on the lower edge (base of the breast), pressing and releasing the thumb and forefinger slightly inwards towards the chest cavity, repeatedly.	Pressing and releasing, pressing and releasing shouldn't hurt. If it hurts, the technique is wrong	
09	Employee/Mother	Gently express the milk to encourage it to come out.	The pressure around the areola must be the same on all sides to ensure that o milk is extracted completely.	Never express on the nipple. Avoid rubbing or sliding your fingers over the skin. The movement of the fingers should be pressing (squeezing and releasing), changing position in a rotating manner.

10	Employee/Mother	Complete emptying of the breasts		0 complete emptying of the breasts enables breastfeeding to be maintained despite the separation of mother and child
11	Employee/Mother	Give o LHOC, immediately after collection, to the recipient, respecting the medical prescription, in terms of volume, route of administration and speed of infusion.	Encourage mothers to offer raw LHOC under the supervision of a health professional. If it is necessary to use an infusion pump, it is recommended that the final administration time, plus the milking time, does not exceed 2 hours.	It promotes bonding, brings mother and child closer together and favours maternal autonomy in caring for the newborn,
12	Employee	Immediately after collection, place the container with the surplus LHOC in the isothermal box prepared in advance with recyclable ice, and send it as quickly as possible in the cold chain to the lactarium, human milk collection centre or human milk bank, for immediate freezing, after cleaning the container with 70% alcohol. Take extra care when identifying and distributing raw milk	0 recyclable ice provides a lower temperature than ordinary ice. Keeping o LHO at refrigeration temperature minimises the proliferation of microorganisms, resulting in a product of greater biological value, with greater bioavailability of calcium and phosphorus.	Respect the cold chain, not leaving the product exposed to the environment. Change gloves after each procedure. If the task is interrupted, change gloves and sanitise hands before restarting.

6.4 Mechanical milking (manual or electric)

Technical Procedures for Milking, Handling and Administering Raw Human Milk Exclusively from Mother to Child in the Neonatal Environment

NOTE: Manual extractor pumps with a rubber pear are not recommended due to the difficulty of

cleaning and sterilising the inside of the pear.

№	AGENT	AQAO	OBSERVATION	COMMENTS
01	Mae	Clean the breasts. a. Clean the breasts with gas and drinking water or; b. Wash the breasts and nipples with running drinking water or; Use human milk itself after the first jets have been eliminated.	It reduces the risk of contamination and also aims to minimise the occurrence of scaling.	Do not use soap or any other type of sanitising product. Do not use creams or ointments with moisturising properties.
02	Employee	Make it available: A. Manual human milk pump or electric, with coupler and sterile storage container. B. Inert and indecisively sterile container with a wide mouth and a screwable plastic lid that allows perfect closure, easy to clean and resistant to the sterilisation process, with a volume compatible with the mother's milk production, with a label to be filled in.		
03	Employee	Provide a support table, previously sanitised in accordance with the protocol adopted by the Institution's ICHR.		
04	Employee/Mother	Massage the breasts as described in item 6.1.		Teaching massage techniques
05	Employee/Mother	Homeexpression softening the areola		

<u>Technical Procedures for Milking, Handling and Administering Raw Human Milk Exclusively from Mother to Child in a </u>Neonatal <u>Setting</u>

№	AGENT	AQAO	OBSERVATION	COMMENTS
06	Employee/Mother	Discard the first jets or drops in sterile gauze.	Improves milk quality by reducing microbial contaminants.	
07	Employee	Fill in the label on the refrigerated sterile container already provided with the name of the recipient's mother, the date and time the milking began.	The label must be resistant to humidity and cooling and must not fade when wet.	
08	Employee/Mother	Touch the coupler to the breast, applying gentle pressure		The nipple should be centred.

09	Employee/Mother	Extract the human milk according to the management instructions for each type of pump used and the volume to be milked. At the end of milking, disconnect the pump from the breast.		Position the pump so that the receptacle/milk storage container is facing downwards.
10	Employee/Mother	Open the pump's collection container under a previously sanitised table, according to the instructions, place the LHOC in the cup or sterile syringe for gavage or translation, and give it to the recipient.	Encourage mothers to offer raw LHOC under the supervision of a health professional. If it is necessary to use an infusion pump, it is recommended that the final administration time, added to the milking time, does not exceed 2 hours.	It promotes bonding, brings mother and child closer together and favours maternal autonomy in caring for the newborn.
11	Employee	Immediately after collection, place the container with surplus LHOC in a pre-prepared cool box with recyclable ice and send it as quickly as possible in a cold chain to the lactarium or human milk collection centre, or	0 recyclable ice provides a lower temperature than ordinary ice. Keeping o LHO at the cooling temperature minimises the	Respect the cold chain by not leaving the product exposed to the environment.

<u>Technical Procedures for Milking, Handling and Administering Raw Human Milk Exclusively from Mother to Child in the</u> Neonatal <u>Environment</u>

		human milk bank, for immediate freezing, after cleaning the bottle with 70% alcohol. Take extra care when identifying and distributing raw milk	proliferation of microorganisms, resulting in a product of greater biological value, with greater bioavailability of calcium and phosphorus.	Change gloves after each procedure. If the task is interrupted, change gloves and sanitise hands before restarting.

6.5. Handling Frozen Raw Milk

№	AGENT	AQAO	OBSERVATION	COMMENTS
1	Lactation Officer/BLH/PCLH	Wearing a mask and cap. Hand hygiene according to ICHC standards		
2	Lactation Officer/BLH/PCLH	Immediately after collection, place the container in a previously prepared cool box with recyclable ice, or in a fridge exclusively for LHO.	0 recyclable ice provides a lower temperature than ordinary ice. Keeping o LHO at	Respect the cold chain by not leaving the product exposed to the environment.

		Take extra care when identifying and distributing raw milk	refrigeration temperature minimises the proliferation of microorganisms, resulting in a product of greater biological value, with greater bioavailability of calcium and phosphorus.	Change gloves after each procedure. If the task is interrupted, change gloves and sanitise hands before restarting.
3	Lactation Officer/BLH/PCLH	Omilk should be transported to the aolactario, human milk bank or PCLH as quickly as possible, maintaining a cold chain with a temperature of around 0°C.	The maximum, minimum and current temperatures of the equipment intended for	The hospital service must have equipment for

Technical Procedures for Milking, Handling and Administering Raw Human Milk Exclusively from Mother to Child in a Neonatal Environment

		of 5^{5} C. Bottles storing breastmilk must be sanitised with 70% alcohol before entering the lactarium or milk bank through a ticket window. LHOC that is not supplied immediately must be labelled in the Neonatal Unit with the date of collection, time, mother's name and sent to the lactarium or HMB, where it will be stored in a freezer exclusively for raw milk, the temperature of which must be < -3^{5} C. The maximum freezing time for raw milk is 15 days.	The storage of LHO must be checked and recorded on instruments designed for this purpose.	exclusively for the storage of LHO. Stocking must be carried out and organised in such a way as to guarantee the identification of the products and avoid the mis-supply of milk.
4	Employee Lactario/BLH/PCLH	Defrosting: a) sanitise your hands and get dressed in the changing room or barrier changing room; b) pour water into a clean bain-marie (change daily or whenever necessary); c) calibrate the water bath to reach a temperature of 40^{5} C (defrosting must be carried out in the water bath); d) after the water bath has reached a temperature of 40^{5} C, remove the LHO vials from the freezer to be thawed;		

		e) place the flasks in the water bath to thaw; f) homogenise the vials with frequent circular movements until the presence of		

		ice stone (approximately 2 cm) in the centre of the jars; g) remove the jars from the water bath and place them in a cooler with water and recyclable ice until serving time or place the jars immediately in a dedicated refrigerator (which should be at a maximum temperature of 5^{5} C) until serving time.		
5	Employee Lactario/BLH/PCLH	Portioning or fractionation: This procedure must be carried out in an exclusive area for this purpose, with sealed windows or protected by millimetre screens when necessary. Doors must be kept closed. *Using a Bunsen burner* or laminar flow hood a) sanitise your hands and wear a mask, cap and goggles in the changing room or barrier changing room; b) sanitise benches with smooth, easy-to-sanitise surfaces using 70% alcohol or a product standardised by the ICHR; cover with a sterile field; c) separate all the labels with the information from the nutritionist's or doctor's prescription (with the newborn's identification), bed, hospitalisation unit, volume and time);		

Technical Procedures for Milking, Handling and Administering Raw Human Milk Exclusively from Mother to Child in the Neonatal Environment

		d) separate all the previously sterilised utensils, which will be used in proportional quantities to the needs; e) Observe the prescription and separate the vials to be used or syringes (when offered by infusion pump or gavage). f) light the Bunsen burner*. In the case of a laminar flow hood - check how long before the start of the procedure it should be switched on for proper operation; g) Sanitise your hands again and dress in a long-sleeved cloak. Wear sterile gloves; h) bring the bottle to the flame field or laminar flow hood, shake the bottle lightly with circular movements and fractionate the milk according to the prescribed volume, in containers suitable for storing human milk (measuring cup) and/or disposable syringe in the flame field or inside the hood. i) If you use a syringe сото meter, you should change the syringe with each bottle; j)cap the appropriate containers for storing human milk at each filling, so that they are tightly sealed, and label them with the appropriate identification tags; syringes should be served with appropriate caps, such as *COMB RED,* never with needles.		

		k) Write down on a spreadsheet the		

		number of aliquots for each nursing mother; l) store the containers of human milk in a dedicated refrigerator, maintaining a temperature of up to 5[5] C, until the moment of distribution; m) send all materials used for washing and sterilisation; n) at the predetermined distribution times, heat the aliquots (bagged individually to prevent water from entering the containers) in a water bath to approximately 36[5] C and send to the Neonatal Unit for administration; o) observe transport precautions, which must be carried out in isothermal boxes, sanitised with 70% alcohol (remembering that the milk is heated to 365C)		

7. General Considerations

№	AGENT	AQAO	OBSERVATION	COMMENTS
1	Neonatal unit employee	Receiving the isothermal boxes in the neonatal unit.	Check the temperature of the isothermal box.	
2	Neonatal unit employee	Check the identification label on the milk received - mother's name, NB, volume to be administered.		
3	Neonatal unit employee	Take to the NB's bed		
4	Neonatal unit employee	Check the time of the diet prescription.	Check the route of administration: oral route -	

Technical Procedures for Milking, Handling and Administering Raw Human Milk Exclusively from Mother to Child in a Neonatal Setting

			translactation (in the presence of the speech therapist or with the technical team), cup, gastric or enteral tube by gavage or infusion pump.	

	Neonatal unit employee	Handle the container in which the milk is stored - always wearing a glove.	If the patient is in contact isolation - observe the other protective items. Follow the ICHR routine.	
5		Cup: handle with procedure glove, position NB and perform the unit technique.		
6	Neonatal unit worker or mother, under supervision	Simple gavage: handle with procedure gloves. Check that the size of the tube is appropriate for the diet, that the tube is correctly positioned and securely attached. Attach the syringe to the distal part of the tube. Remove the embolus and allow the milk to flow down by gravity. The milk should not be administered by pushing on the embolus. Once the milk has flowed in. Remove the syringe and close the tube.	If there is any doubt about the correct location of the tube (the outer part is longer than usual) - change the tube. Larger calibre tubes should not be used for patients on a diet. Larger calibre tubes are used for gas decompression. Gastric residue is no longer checked. Therefore, attach the syringe and start administering the diet (by gravity).	
7	Neonatal unit employee	Diet in infusion pump: handle with procedure gloves. Attach the syringe to the infusion pump and the syringe nozzle to the distal part of the tube. Check the infusion rate programmed in the	The maximum time that milk can be infused is 2 hours. If the prescription calls for a longer infusion time, we must	

		and set the parameter on the pump's display.	change the syringe and receive a new aliquot of milk. So that no fat is lost from the wall of the syringe, we can homogenise the milk from time to time - just remove it from the pump and rub the syringe	

			between both hands.	

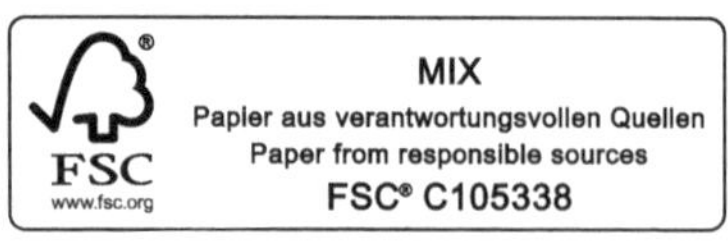

Printed by Books on Demand GmbH, Norderstedt / Germany